Alopecia & Wellness

How I Got My Hair Back Treatment Free

Molly Vazquez

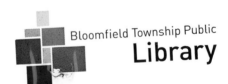

Bloomfield Township Public
Library

1099 Lone Pine Road
Bloomfield Township, Michigan 48302
(248) 642-5800 | www.btpl.org

Introduction

I was thinking too hard about alopecia and how to cure

it, instead of what it actually was. "What is alopecia and what is

it doing to the inside of my body?" That was the question I had

to ask myself, instead of the obvious "I'm bald, so what

treatment can grow my hair back?" That question only led down

the same miserable path of my bald reality.

Let's be honest. The real reason you're reading this book is

because you are like I was: sick of having no hair and tired of

feeling like the cue ball on the pool table. Most likely, just

reading the word *alopecia* gives you a knot in your chest and a

lump in your throat, because you are so emotionally attached to

this disease. Or maybe finding this book gave you some relief

for once, because someone is recognizing your "biggest flaw

and biggest pain." Those two feelings were the only ones that were real to me when I had to live with alopecia. Any other feelings were just a cover for how hurt I was underneath my hairless skin.

So yes, I know how you feel, and that gives me the right to say with you: *alopecia sucks!*

Now that I've gotten the obvious out there, I can tell you what this book is about. I share my story with alopecia and how I got my hair back treatment free. I will not get too medical in this book, or make this book so difficult to read that you get bored and toss it aside. After all, as a reader with alopecia, you really just want to know how I got my hair back. I can say I did *not* get my hair back from treatments, poisonous shots in my head, or anything that's touted as a cure. If you're wondering if this is about eating better, the simple answer is yes! But there is more to it than eating better. It's a lifestyle change as a whole.

Let me break this down: alopecia is an autoimmune disease.

"Disease" is an effect from a body being unbalanced. The hint is in the name: dis-ease. When I decided to "let food by thy medicine," it was to heal my body for the sake of my health, not my hair. If I had tried to conquer alopecia solely by focusing on how to get my hair back and not my health, I would still resemble a gerbil running on its wheel, chasing nothing. I chose to look beyond the cage and consider what my disease really was about. My body was yelling at me to get healthier!

My healthy routines are simple and they are what's real. My body is real. The fact that my hair fell out from an immune-combating disease is real. Health is something I had to learn to take seriously. Besides, what would have happened next if my body continued being compromised? I cleaned up my lifestyle so that nothing could damage my body anymore, and let my body heal naturally.

In simple words—steady, essential routines equal a clean, harm-free body.

Alopecia is an autoimmune disease.

Definition of an autoimmune disease:

Auto means: self

Immune means: to protect against something
disagreeable

Disease means state of imbalance (dis-ease)

If you put all those together so they make sense, the
body's immune systems fails to protect itself, putting the body at
risk and out of balance.

An autoimmune disease is an illness that occurs when the body's
tissues are attacked by the body's own immune system. The
immune system is a complex organization within the body that
is designed to "seek and destroy" invaders of the body,
including infectious agents. Patients with autoimmune diseases
frequently have unusual antibodies circulating in their blood

which target their bodies' tissues.

In the case of alopecia, the tissue is attacked by the hair follicle (called papilla), the structure from which hair grows. Alopecia can affect any person at any age. Approximately 200 million people in the world have alopecia. In the Unites States alone, approximately 4 million people are affected.

Here are the different kinds of alopecia:

Alopecia areata refers to hair loss that occurs in round patches. (These patches can appear anywhere on the body.)

Alopecia totalis refers to the loss of hair on the scalp. As the name suggests, alopecia totalis is total baldness.

Alopecia universalis results in the loss of hair from a person's entire body.

Alopecia barbae affects only men, and refers to the loss of hair in the beard area.

Alopecia happens when the hair loss is accompanied by the appearance of scaly patches on the skin.

Anagen effluvium is hair loss that is commonly associated with chemotherapy and with taking certain kinds of medication. In anagen effluvium, the hair falls out in patches, although it grows back as soon as the chemotherapy or the consumption of the affecting medications stops.

Telogen effluvium is also called temporary hair loss. It happens when the amount of hair being shed is more than normal and the hair visibly thins.

Androgenetic alopecia is considered hereditary. It is also known as male pattern baldness, although it can also affect women. In androgenetic alopecia, the hair on the scalp turns nearly transparent before falling off.

Scarring alopecia happens when the skin is scarred by

the hair shedding.

Traction alopecia is due to a person's hair being pulled too much, sometimes from styling and sometimes from personal habits. The excessive pulling can discourage the hair follicles from developing new cells for new hair.

Having alopecia wasn't a death sentence, but just because I wasn't dying didn't mean I wasn't sick. When I finally understood that, I realized I had to focus on my health, not my hair. First I knew that what was harming me on the inside had to come out. The only way to do that, my common sense told me, was to eliminate the old food I had eaten. I figured that if I started to eat healthier foods, then the old harmful food would be eliminated and my body could begin to heal.

And that's just what happened.

This was my journey with alopecia.

My Story

In 2001, when I was seven, my family moved into a new home in a nice town in Massachusetts. The town was quaint and inviting, perfect for middle-class families. My brother and I are fourteen months apart in age. My mom had him start school late, so we could enter the first grade together. We quickly made friends with some kids who happened to be neighbors. In the middle of my neighborhood was a park and a baseball field. All the kids met there every day, playing baseball and riding our bikes until dinnertime. In my spare time I enjoyed drawing and writing. Creativity runs in my family, and there are some amazing artists on both sides. I was lucky enough to get that creativity gene. My parents didn't believe in video games, so to entertain ourselves, my brother and I had to use our imaginations. My mom's favorite quote was, "Boredom creates creativity."

My brother and I played in baseball and basketball leagues for many years. Everyone always laughed when they saw how good I was, the only girl on the boys' teams. I was a petite child with the flair of a tomboy.

By the time we were in the fourth grade, my mom realized my brother and I weren't happy in school. She asked us if we wanted to be homeschooled. We looked at each other, and I remember saying, "Are you kidding?" Honestly, I had never felt so relieved. Agreeing to homeschooling was one of the best decisions of my life. Being able to study independently took a huge weight off my chest. I could actually read what I had to read without being on a time limit. Louis and I felt like we were the luckiest kids on earth.

In 2006, one year later, when I was twelve years old, I was in the bathroom doing the same routine I did every day: complain about brushing my teeth, take a shower, and brush my hair. As I was brushing my hair, I noticed an itching at the back of my head. It was the most irritating feeling. It felt like my hair was brushing up against the back of my scalp. Finally I found the exact area that was bothering me and noticed there was a bald spot about the size of a quarter. I didn't think much of this discovery, but I called my mom in anyway. Even though she didn't show me that she was worried, I still knew she wasn't as laid back as I was about that little bald spot. She just said, "Hmm?", tilted her head, and then said, "Let's give it a few days. If it gets any worse, we'll call the doctor."

Every day after that, hair was *everywhere*: on my pillow, in my sheets, all over the bathtub after my shower, with clumps in the drain. It didn't take long for my mom to realize it was time to call the doctor.

She made an appointment with our physician, and he saw us that day. The doctor took pictures of my head for my file and gave my mom a dermatologist's name and number. He also told me that when I was an adult, I would have the option of getting cortisone shots that weren't necessarily going to work. Since I had an autoimmune disease, I was not going to do any more harm that hadn't already been done by using a poisonous treatment that hadn't been proven to do much. Oh, and I got a name for my new condition: alopecia areata, an autoimmune disease that can cause the rapid shedding of hair in patchlike bald spots.

There are several different kinds of alopecia, and they are all pretty similar. Meaning, they all are autoimmune diseases and they all make the sufferers lose hair, either complete baldness or just bald spots, and either all over the body or just on the head. What I know for sure is that they all made me go through hell and back. If you have one form of alopecia, it means you can develop a different form of it. You can lose your hair in patchy bald spots (alopecia areata) at any time, and then randomly have alopecia totalis and lose all of your scalp hair. Let's just say alopecia wages a constant battle with your appearance and your psyche.

***

The second we left the physician's office, my mom phoned the dermatologist, whom our doctor had called "the best known." Mom booked an appointment, but couldn't get in for six months.

I just kept losing more and more hair. Every couple of months, my head was like a pizza with more slices being taken out of it. I wore a baseball cap whenever I left the house, hoping no one noticed that I had only a couple strands of hair. After a while, it got too obvious, so my mom and I went to a beauty store to see what my options were for fake hair.

Of course they showed me wigs. Not just any wigs, but the itchiest kind of fake hair you can imagine. I tried one on and it was unbelievably irritating. Not to mention that it looked like woven cotton had given birth to a broom. There was no way I was going to wear that nest, so I thought it would be a good idea to take hair extensions and glue them to the inside of my favorite hat. It looked like I really had hair underneath, but it still added another deep sigh of melancholy to my life. I mean, hair extensions were the highlight of my day?

Six months went by slowly, and the day of hope finally arrived. My appointment to go see the dermatologist had come. He told me the same things my doctor had, though he went into a little more depth. I found out that since I was young and had already lost my hair, the chances were slim to none that I would ever see a strand of hair again. I could also expect my eyebrows, eyelashes, and other body hair to fall out.

So there I was, twelve years old and destined to have no hair at all! Like the awkward stage wasn't bad enough! Waiting six miserable months just to have my disease confirmed and explained in slow motion was not what I'd had in mind from "the best known" dermatologist. Sitting in that waiting room for an hour having every excited emotion you can name, I had believed I actually was going to have a normal childhood. Instead, it was the worst day of my life. I felt my spirit burst into a million pieces. What was even worse was that the dermatologist expressed no sympathy for me at all. He told me the bad news nonchalantly. When he walked in the room and said all the things I already knew and gave no advice, I just sat in the same paused position, staring at the wall. His words went in and out, loud and then quiet, like sound waves.

I walked out of there knowing I was going to be the different girl my whole life. The days of my perfect hair and bangs were over; the nights when I just threw my hair up in a messy bun were over. That day at the dermatologist's confirmed that being a hairless girl was my new life.

Oh, but since I was pretty much bald at that point, he did say something I didn't know: "You have alopecia totalis."

As we walked out of the office, my mom acted like she still had hope for me, but I knew we were thinking the same thing— "Now what?" I couldn't accept living with this, but I had no clue what to do. I really had no information, and the doctors I had relied on for some answers merely verified what I knew and were really no help. I was going to have to deal with it myself, and hopefully something good would come my way. But every day from then on, I didn't have a thought that didn't whisper worry about my hair.

***

I quit baseball because it was getting too rough for a small girl, switching over to softball. I still played basketball too, but I had to play wearing my hat with the glued extensions. In order to do that, my mom had to tell the coach about my condition so I could wear the hat during games. Coach Comak was so understanding and such a nice guy, and was always supportive of me. Although I couldn't play as well as I used to, because I was afraid someone would knock my hat off, I still loved basketball. I did my best and acted like no one knew I was the only one on the court with a hat on. Sports were a way for me to remain myself and feel normal. Since I was homeschooled, they were also a way for me to still see the kids from my old school and make new friends. Every time I made a shot and it went into the basket, it was so satisfying, and I needed that. I couldn't just stay home in a bubble crying about what I'd lost.

I remember one particular game had three seconds left. I had the ball on the other end of the court. I turned around and hooked the ball really fast, not evening thinking I would make it in. The buzzer sounded and I started to walk off the court, but then realized the whole gym was dead quiet and no one was moving. I looked around, wondered what was going on. A friend ran up to me and said, "You just made that shot!"

Another game did not go so well. I was ready to play, but my coach had forgotten to inform the referee that I had to wear my hat. I got to start out with the ball, but the ref blew his whistle and in front of everyone told me to take my hat off. I couldn't even talk and was so embarrassed, I felt like I had swallowed my chest. The coach just said I couldn't take my hat off, and the ref said it was okay.

I'm not the kind of girl who cares what others think of her, but this was the one thing I was always afraid of. Just anyone mentioning my hair reflected on how normal I wasn't and how much of a nightmare my reality actually was.

***

My family has always been fortunate enough to take a vacation once a year. We all look forward to it, starting with the day we plan it. Whenever I am having a bad day, I just picture myself on our vacation, regardless of how far away it is. Six months, three months, two weeks, I still get butterflies.

Now that I had no hair, I thought about our yearly vacation more than ever. It felt good that the people I would see were people I would never see again. I wanted to be as free as possible, just let go and forget about my alopecia. I decided not to wear my hat with the extensions in the airport, but a bandana instead. The whole airport adventure was just a bunch of people coming up to my parents and asking if I had cancer, if I was sick, if I was going to be okay. I was fortunate not to have cancer, but that didn't mean I was happy. Everywhere I went I was being reminded about something I just wanted to end. I felt like I was in a fish tank and people wouldn't stop tapping on the glass. I didn't let that ruin my vacation, though. I just decided to push it out of my mind and try to enjoy the trip as much as I could.

***

A few weeks later, my mom was getting her hair done. Her hair dresser said that a friend of hers went to a place that specialized in hair loss. My mom called and found out that since I was under eighteen, I could get a free hairpiece that was valued at $1500. I would be able to customize the color, and they would measure my head so it was comfortable. Not to mention that it was made of real hair. When it came in, a hairdresser there would style it the way I wanted.

21

When the day came for me to be fitted for the hairpiece, I couldn't help but be excited about getting my new hair. On top of that, my grandma was visiting. I don't know why I didn't understand what it meant to get a hairpiece. I thought they were going to grow my hair follicles somehow and attach extensions. I've always had a creative mind, so I thought up all sorts of different ways this hair was going to be attached to my head. I thought this was the solution, and I wasn't going to be bald my whole life.

Sitting in the salon chair at that hair club as they measured my head was an experience. It was a very creative process, I must say. They put plastic wrap on my scalp and then stuck wide clear tape around the crown of my head, molding the plastic wrap to the size and shape of my skull. They sent the mold out to make the custom hairpiece so that it would fit as well and as comfortably as possible. This place was no joke. They were literally custom hairpiece makers. I still wasn't connecting the dots that I was being fitted for a wig.

After they finished measuring me, we made an appointment to come back for the final fitting. On that day, when they put my new hairpiece on and tightly attached it to my head with double-sided adhesive tape, I almost burst into tears.

The stylist was so happy. You could tell hairdressing was her passion. My hairpiece that she styled was her creation. She pretty much did her own thing with my hairpiece, and I looked like an eighties beauty pageant contestant. She was trying so hard to make it look nice for me, I couldn't say anything. I didn't want to say, (after all she did), that I was a tomboy who preferred straight hair with straight bangs, like I'd had my whole life. My mom saw the look on my face when we left and she said she'd fix it when we got home.

I was so grateful that I could walk out my door without a

baseball hat on, and I thought my days in disguise were over. I had just got another disguise, though, something that I could hide under. My cousin had been at the salon with my mom and I, and she was so supportive while I was so embarrassed. All I had been talking about was how I was going to get my "new hair." I had told my grandma, my cousins, my parents and brother how I was looking forward to being me again. Now I felt like a joke. I had been painting a picture in my head for a while, but reality had hit me with not just a brick, but the whole building.

The weird part for me was going home and everyone still knowing me, when I didn't even recognize myself. I felt like a distorted version of me, and I had done nothing to get myself in this position.

**

My friend Stacy from our softball team invited me to her birthday party at her home. The whole team was there and it was really fun. When they all decided to go swimming in her pool, I acted like I just wanted to put my feet in the water. I'd been told I couldn't get my hairpiece wet. Everyone called to me, "Oh, c'mon, Molly! C'mon!" They all were having a good time and I wanted to join them, so I jumped in. I figured, how bad could my hairpiece be if it got wet? Actually, while I was in the pool and the hairpiece was soaking wet, it was fine and the hair lay right down. I was laughing and completely let go, relieved that I could be myself. When we all got out and dried off, I felt my hair shrinking into a tight knot. I ran into the bathroom. Luckily my mom had stayed since she was friends with Stacy's mom, and she helped me take the hairpiece off. She shampooed and conditioned it five times. Then I put it on and she blow-dried it

25

for me. There was way too much chlorine in the pool and my hair couldn't take it.

On another summer day, it was so unbelievably hot and my friend Erika thought it was a perfect beach day. My mom and her mom agreed to take us. I didn't think going into the ocean with my hairpiece on would be a problem. I thought it just couldn't handle chlorine.

It was such a fun day at the beach. Erika and I were playing in the water, and out of nowhere a huge wave swept over us. I was completely underwater, and my head dug into the sandy bottom. When I got up, I felt sand everywhere you can imagine. We ran out and grabbed out towels. As I was rubbing the sand off me, I felt sand slide out from underneath my hairpiece. I told my mom to come with me to the bathroom, and once again we had to take my "hair" off and remove all the sand. Even though we got the sand out, I didn't have any products to clean the hair or blow-dry it so that it looked real and normal. I just had to go out to my friend and act like nothing had happened, like my hair didn't look ratty and unattached from my head.

Slowly everyone started connecting the dots that my hair wasn't real. After that, people either started treating me differently or I didn't hear from them again. On the other hand, I got really close with my two cousins, Anna and Alexa. I felt comfortable with them since they didn't judge me about having no hair. They came over to my house a lot, and every time they came over, I got my hairpiece all ready and done up. My mom thought it was ridiculous for me to keep putting my hairpiece on, especially since it was summer. Sometimes my cousins would sleep over too, not for just one night, but days.

One day, in front of my cousins, my mom said, "Molly, just take off your hairpiece for them."

My cousins smiled and encouraged me, saying that it was okay.

I couldn't do it. I was insistent about never showing anyone my bald head. My mom took me into the bathroom, saying, "You have to, Molly. It will be good for you."

I took off my hair, but then I burst into tears, saying that I didn't want to. I had the biggest knot in my chest. My mom picked me up, and I cried against her shoulder. She opened the bathroom door and carried me out. Anna and Alexa ran over and patted my back, saying how pretty I was.

I was so ashamed. I asked my mom for one of my hats—without extensions. Once my hat was on, I wiped my tears away and stood up, relieved that the big reveal was over. That was really therapeutic for me. Now every time my cousins came and slept over, I didn't have to have my hairpiece on all day and night. When we went out, I'd throw my hair on.

***

One of the stories my mom always tells certain people is about when I was getting prepped for braces and had to wear a headgear at night. One night I had a nightmare and went into my paren'ts room. Picture a girl with a bald head and headgear wrapped around her face. I asked if I could sleep with them. My mom said, "No, Molly, you have to sleep in your own bed," but my dad said, "Oh, come on, look at her." They let me sleep with them.

***

My family moved north, still living in Massachusetts but near New Hampshire. This time we upgraded our home from middle class to upper class. We met a few different families in our new neighborhood. One couple, Christina and Robert, had two children. Carissa was about my age, and her little brother Noah was two. My mom needed a new hairdresser, and Christine did hairdressing on the side. At first, I went with my mom and hung out with Carissa while my mom got her hair done. I only had a few friends and the number had been slowly decreasing, so it felt good to be starting fresh in my new town. I loved playing with Carissa's little brother. Carissa had to watch him most of the time while Christina was doing hair. Most little kids tended to like me, and Noah was no exception. He gave me a nickname: Mo-mo. Since I was homeschooled, Christina would sometimes invite me over while Carissa was in school since Noah loved me. She and I would always laugh and have a good time.

While I had alopecia, I enjoyed kids and their innocent minds, and most adults understood and were genuinely caring. It was refreshing and something I definitely needed at that time. Eventually, when my mom and Christina became friends, she told Christina about my alopecia and my hairpiece. I didn't really mind when adults knew, but I was worried about Carissa finding out, or any of my other friends.

One day Noah pulled my hair. He had the tightest grip and would not let go. Carissa and her friend Lindsey were there as well, and they watched me. Since my hairpiece was held on by adhesive tape, you can imagine the pain I was in as Noah yanked on the hair. All I could think was, *God, please make this kid let go.* Outwardly I was calm. I looked him in the eyes and said nicely, "Let go, Noah. Let go, Noah," while trying to smile. My eyes were watering with every tug, and he still would not let go. I felt like my head was being cut around the rim with a steak knife. Finally I pinched his hand a little. He left go and burst into tears. I slowly walked into the bathroom and let the tears from the pain fall. After that I wore my hair in a ponytail when I knew I would be watching him.

Carissa and I were become close, and I consider her one of my best friends. She invited me to a sleepover at her house to celebrate her birthday, along with a few of her friends that I had

met before. The night was going well and I was having such a

good time. We were watching a move when Christina came

upstairs. We paused the movie so she could ask Carissa

something. Christina glanced at the TV, which was fixed on an

unappealing girl with messy hair, and started laughing.

"Look, it's Molly!" she exclaimed. "Hey, Molly, look, it's you."

She said that at least five times, and Carissa yelled at her in

embarrassment, "Stop, Mom!"

I have pride, but I've never had to shove tears so far back into

my eyes before.

I've been stared at, whispered about, pointed at, but I had never

had this happen to me, especially from an adult who was one of

my mom's friends, and one of my older friends as well.

Someone who knew of my condition.

I had always been an independent child, but this episode taught

me why I should remain independent. I learned who my true
friends were, and I could count them on one hand. Carissa was a
good friend. I even brought her back a trophy from Disney
World that said World's Best Friend. I brought Noah a stuffed
Winnie-the-Pooh that I knew he would love.

After a while, though, Christina must have told Carissa about
my alopecia, because she wasn't the same anymore. Every time
she looked at me, she seemed to be thinking of something else.
Probably, *Is that really a wig?* She and her friend Lindsey
started instant messaging me on AIM, bullying me and
provoking fights. We stopped being friends.

A couple of weeks later Carissa called and apologized three
times. I decided to give her another chance. I went over to her
house, and out of nowhere she and her mom started laughing.
They told me how they had seen me with my swim cap on at my
grandfather's pool down the street. That was the last time I saw

them.

How I Felt
Seeing My Hair Fall Out

The feeling of losing my hair, especially that quickly, is indescribable. Being twelve and going through hormonal changes is enough for a child to handle. Add a new traumatic experience to that and, well, it's indescribable. Honestly, there are no words that come close to conveying what I felt. I tried so hard to ignore the inconceivable pain inside my chest and the thoughts that were tearing up my mind.

What bothered me more than not having hair was that my body was doing this to me. Of course my appearance in the mirror sliced away every ounce of confidence I had. The self-attacking disease was an invasion that violated me way past my comfort zone, to my core. With every hair follicle that alopecia released from my head, the emotional lump in my throat grew and salty tears welled in my eyes. The fading glow of my skin was the only residue left of my exterior. I felt like my body had been taken over by a demon, and I had been pushed onto a scary trail that lead into the unknown. I used to be fearless, never let anything get to me. Once I got this disease, every little thing offended me. I started to take everything to heart. My thoughts narrowed onto negative thinking, and people who saw me probably wondered why I looked so miserable.

Even though Mom taught me how to weigh my perspectives with her spot-on observations, she didn't know the dreams that started to grow in me. Alopecia made me feel recognized for the wrong reasons, and that gave me a burning ambition to be recognized one day for the right reasons. I wanted to be noticed for the real me and not the emotions that had pushed me into a place of pain. And not for how weird my hairpiece looked. I wanted to be admired and not made fun of. I wanted to be a role model for girls of all ages, and wanted boys to respect me and be attracted to me. Even with all my negative thinking, I was too stubborn to settle on this disease as a permanent condition, even though that's what doctors said.

As my dreams for recognition and stardom grew, I began breaking through the barrier of all things impossible. I might not have had hair or been my true self in reality, but I had my own secret world of possibilities in my mind. I could visit that world anytime I wanted, to escape from the frustrating reality I was in. In my head was the real me; in my reality was what I had been condemned to live with. I wasn't letting go of the images of stardom, not if my life depended on it.

It didn't help that I was going through puberty when I lost my hair. My appearance seemed to change daily. I was growing into a person I didn't recognize, and I was faced with a huge question: Who am I? I had no idea, and what made it worse was that I had no say in my appearance. I did, at least, have a say over the clothes I wore every day.

At the time, my overall style was influenced by Avril Lavigne. She is a pop/rock singer whose music really hit home with me.

Her lyrics stuck with me, and my favorite is:
Is it enough to love?
Is it enough to breathe? …
Somebody save my life
I'd rather be anything but ordinary please

Not having many friends always led me back to the "happy world" in my mind. In that world, I would daydream about meeting Avril. She was my role model at that time, and it seemed like she was the only one who could put my feelings into words. This dream wouldn't leave my mind. It felt so real! Then one day I got on her website and saw that she was doing a concert in Boston, near where I lived. I could purchase meet and greet tickets! What were the odds of that? Of course my mom said we could go.

I learned then the power of a dream that burns in the gut and takes over the mind. I had planted a seed, and hope and will had watered that seed. Eventually it would become what I had planted. Was I crazy and overthinking, or was I on to something? I wanted to find out, so I tried an even bigger dream. What was it that I wanted more than anything? That was easy: I wanted alopecia to stop taking over my body, and I wanted a recovery that would allow my hair to grow back.

Just that thought was an enormous step toward enlightenment. Okay, so I had planted the seed and hopefully it would grow. Now all I had to do was picture it becoming reality and believe it was going to happen. Deciding to dream big, I pictured myself not just with hair, but with thick hair with highlights, my body radiant with a glow, and myself gorgeous. I wrapped this image around me as if it were a life vest that would keep me from drowning.

I didn't know it at the time, but I was teaching myself the power of vision. All I knew was that I was a depressed bald girl, bored to tears, who was using her creative skills to dream on a remarkable level. This is probably why I'm drawn to celebrities. They start with a dream and never let go of their vision until they achieve it. Even though I didn't have many friends, I had those celebrities on TV, in magazines, and on the Internet, who influenced my life. I learned from the successful. When I finally started making friends again, it was nice to have people to actually talk with, but my ears were still pitched for the inspiration of successful people. It's a bittersweet trait that's a part of me to this day, and it has always helped me push beyond boundaries to what is seen as impossible, to understand who those slim odds are really meant for.

To nurture my dream, I would go to bed at night and picture myself the way I wanted to be. Every time I woke up and nothing had changed, I was a little disappointed but more at ease with that reality. My dream of hair was so strong, I could actually feel my fingers running through my perfect locks. This kept my mind on a positive level. I started following fashion and considered the different hair styles I might want to try when my hair grew in. Why not? What did I have to lose, more hair? I was already bald.

One of the worst aspects of alopecia was that it didn't affect only me. It affected my whole family. I was always an introvert, but then I felt so ugly, with no control over my body, I just shut down. Most days, I would smoosh my face into a pillow and scream out my frustrations. My father, mother and brother felt hopeless right along with me. Whatever I felt, they felt.

My brother Louie and I are best friends, and since we were

being homeschooled together, we were even closer. Louie and I have a bond that other kids never could understand. When I lost my hair, Louie didn't know what to say. No one knew what to say. Everyone just left me alone and tried to overlook the elephant in the room.

What killed me at the time was knowing how much pain my mom, dad, and brother were in because of what was happening to me. We all lost our zest for life together. They saw my sense of humor turn into crying day after day. My free spirit was gone, and I adopted a new expression—a frown carved on my face. Despite that, my family never treated me any differently.

I could tell my dad didn't know what to say. To watch his little girl's life change for the worse, could his be enjoyable? Knowing that while he was at work I was home crying, traumatized by something he couldn't make better, was painful. How could he say, It's going to be okay, when no one knew if it

would be okay or not? I knew at the time he wished he would
tickle me until I laughed so hard, but that was a temporary high.
As for my mom, she was there to witness my first bald spot. She
was the one who made the appointment to go see the doctors.
She made sure she kept her own head on straight so I would
have a role model. She kept the whole family afloat in the worst
times. She continued homeschooling Louie and I, and she made
sure we both got equal attention from her. Life went on because
of her. Even though half of me was shut down, She kept the
other half of me running like a computer in screen-saver mode.
She wouldn't let me shut down completely. I'm sure that when I
screamed she wanted to scream, but she knew she had to be my
rock and refuge. She always kept me thinking on a higher level
when she said, "There has to be another way out of this disease.
You don't have to have it your whole life. That can't just be it."
My mother has the young mind of a dreamer, and she helped me

to learn to dream big, without limitation, and without doubting myself. She taught me to predict my own outcome and to never settle on something I didn't want to settle on.

Chiropractic

My mom made friends with a couple, Marge and George, who lived on the same street as my grandfather. His house was around the corner from ours, and since we walked our dogs to his house all the time, we eventually met Marge. She was a tall gray-haired woman past her middle years. My mom is very charismatic, and Marge was the same. Those two could talk for hours, so it's no surprise she and Marge instantly became friends.

When they took a walk together one day, Marge mentioned a Gonstead chiropractor she saw every week, and how grateful she was for the practice of chiropractic. My mom told her she had injured her shoulder a while ago at the gym and it was still bothering her. Marge invited her to a couple of workshops, where chiropractors educated attendees on the importance of a healthy spine and the amazing results that followed chiropractic adjustments.

My mom went to a workshop and came home speechless for all the information she'd learned. She announced that we were all going to see a chiropractor, and that she'd made appointments for us to have our spines X-rayed.

I went with my mom when she got hers done. When the chiropractor displayed her X-ray, he highlighted swollen or irritated parts of her spine. I didn't think much of it. I was twelve and had bigger problems. I just wanted to go out to lunch after the appointment. I didn't understand how chiropractic worked. I didn't see how this back cracking called "adjustments" was going to help anything, or how it could be important. My X-ray also revealed swelling and irritation in certain areas.

The chiropractor didn't know about my alopecia until my first

adjustment. I had to lie down on his mechanical chiropractic

bed. I hadn't been in the mood to wear my hairpiece, so I was

wearing my hat with the extensions. He told me to lie on my

stomach and flip my hat backward so I could put my head down.

I froze and quickly looked at my mom.

"She can't," she said, and glared at the doctor as if to say, "I'll

tell you later."

She told him after he had finished my adjustment. He said, "I've

never heard of someone with alopecia getting their hair back

from this, but nothing's impossible. Adjustments won't hurt."

I didn't exactly have great confidence in chiropractic when I

heard that, but my mom had an instinct that we were onto

something. She thought this might be a good path. I wanted an

answer too, and I was sick of waiting. I had been totally bald for

a year and half of my left eyebrow was now gone.

***

My mom continued to go to the workshops, sometimes

with Marge and sometimes on her own. Every time she came

home, she taught us all about what she'd learned. For example,

getting your spine adjusted was just as important a routine as

brushing your teeth. The spine can be misaligned, causing

illness and disease.

Our spines are connected to our nerves, and our nerves are

connected to our organs and, of course, our nervous systems.

The nervous system helps the body heal when it is sick. When

the spine is misaligned, chiropractors can locate nerve

interference in the spine. Everybody has nerve interference. It

affects different people in different ways, but in general nerve

interference blocks the passage for the body to heal itself. So

when a chiropractor corrects interference, every spinal

adjustment promotes natural healing abilities and boosts the immune system.

Learning all of that, my mom kept educating herself, feeding her instincts. She had such a strong feeling that this was the right path, a piece of the puzzle.

My family and I have being going to a chiropractor once a week for five years now. My father broke his back years ago, and he's always had pain. Once he started to get adjusted, he immediately felt light. He'd never been into painkillers or surgery because he knew those would just cover his pain and not necessarily fix him. Adjustments completely corrected what was wrong, targeting what the pain was connected to. To this day he still feels amazing. Chiropractic allows him to keep up with our family construction business, which he's been involved in for nearly thirty years.

My brother started working in the business when he was eighteen. With such a physical job, it only makes sense for him to be adjusted as well, to keep his spine aligned and to keep him completely healthy. My mom had a pain in her neck, through her shoulder, and down her back. Before she started seeing a chiropractor, I can't remember a night when she didn't have an ice pack glued to her upper back. Now, so long as she gets adjusted, she has no pain.

Our weekly adjustments have helped each of us in unique ways. By having the problems in our spines located and corrected, our bodies have been allowed to heal.

Chiropractic really opened my family's eyes to healing the body. I started to educate myself more about healing, and how everyday routines have a huge impact on our health and our bodies.

Mental

"We cannot solve our problems with the same kind of thinking that we used when we created them". -Albert Einstein

At thirteen years olds, I was bald with alopecia totalis, with half of one eyebrow gone. The next level, alopecia universalis, was starting to hit me. Alopecia universalis means that every single hair on my body could fall out. My eyebrows were my only facial feature that made me look somewhat normal. Without my eyebrows, my hairpiece would look completely fake. What was I supposed to do, pencil on eyebrows every day? What if my eyelashes fell out? I would have to glue on fake eyelashes to protect my eyes? A whole 'nother list of worries were added to my life! What did I do to deserve this?

I had no idea what I would do if my family weren't so great and supportive. The only positive thoughts in my head most days were, "When's lunch so I can eat my feelings"; and, Thank God I'm homeschooled so I don't have to face kids' opinions of my appearance. Adults, I'd found, were more understanding of disease, while most kids would put me in the Twilight Zone with their mean comments and the way they would exclude me. If I'd had to go to school every day, I would have felt so isolated.

I saw everyone chasing his or her dreams and goals, while I was forced to stop and face what was real. Reality hits us when the unpredictable happens, and I definitely had never seen myself with no hair. I might have been young when I learned that, but I also knew it was up to me to turn my disease into a learning experience, not a life-draining circumstance. Only I could stop myself from my goal of getting my hair back. No one cared more about my disease than I did, and it wasn't up to anyone to cry over what I'd lost. I developed the attitude: If it is to be, it is up to me. Besides, crying a river was only going to drown me.

***

We moved again two years later, when I was fourteen, into another upper-class neighborhood just a couple of towns over. The house was new but had been built to have a Victorian look. Everyone in the neighborhood was so nice. Their personalities matched their amazing homes aswell. My brother and I immediately made friends. I can't tell you the last time I had friends that were this nice and genuine. It felt good to start fresh again.

I started listening to a Joel Osteen CD. Osteen is a pastor at Lakewood Church in Houston, Texas, and the author of best-selling books and audio CDs. When I first listened to his CD, I pictured him motivating a small crowd of people in a small historic church in Texas. When I went online to see what this guy was all about, I couldn't believe how big is $100 million church is.

He speaks about God and thinking positive, and how you can overcome anything. My favorite quote of his is, "Are you a victim, or are you a victor?" That saying has had the biggest impact on my life. I didn't realize at the time that I was acting like a victim of my own life, when it was up to me to wake and smell the roses. Only I could pull myself out of my rut. I had to learn to appreciate the positive things that were around me, instead of focusing on the negatives or a past I couldn't change. Even thought my family doesn't attend church, I consider us on the spiritual side. We choose to be nice and understanding of other people, while not letting them affect who we are as people. The Osteen CD made me consider the impact my thoughts and actions had on my life every day. I had to believe I was going to get where I wanted to be. I could only do that with a more forward approach to how I went about achieving my goals. The last thing I needed were negative thoughts eating that image away.

When I looked in the mirror before, all I saw was a girl with a wig. Now I started seeing myself for the first time in years. I don't think I'd looked at my face without dwelling on my wig or bald head first. Just by changing my thoughts, all of those worried whispers were going away because I chose not to listen to them anymore.

I had so much energy now from being happy, I started walking my dogs with my mom and exercising more. I hadn't felt that free since before I lost my hair, when all I did was ride my bike and play sports.

From what I've observed, most alopecia victims try to treat the outside of their heads and wonder why it's not working. Even the dermatologist just explained my head and hair. Everything I heard about alopecia was just babbling about how horrible it is to lose your hair, hair, hair, hair! I took a different approach. I

changed my perspective on the way I thought about alopecia.

From then on I didn't think about my hair or what I had for hair.

I didn't even think about the hairpiece I had to wear around my

friends. For me, a change of mind was a change of life. What I

know now is that negative thoughts tend to have a domino

effect. Thinking clearly was a choice I had to make every single

time I thought it was up to me to control not just what I thought,

but *how* I thought. Regardless, I was still a young teenager with

whirlwind emotions and a long list of reasons to be moody.

I have to put on a wig, God? Why me? The worst thing for any

girl to go through? I'm just trying to grow into the pretty girl I

know I can be. But I have to put on a wig every day or look at

my unsightly head? It's hard enough to make friends out there

and then to keep them once they find out about my big 'flaw.' I

watch girls my age on dates with boys at the movies and I think that will never be me. Nobody will accept an ugly girl.

Those were the thought I had for years every night before I went

to bed. Some nights, if I was lucky, I wouldn't cry. It wasn't

easy getting rid of these thoughts, but I did. I just kept trying to

notice the great things in life and pushing those negative

thoughts aside.

I hadn't realized how much the negativity was draining me.

Sometimes you simply need a pick-me-up to turn not just your

day around, but your life.

Worrying will set you back! Think of this analogy:

It's like when couples want to get pregnant so, so, so badly but

they're full of stress and worry every time they try! Than once

they finally give up or take a break from trying, BOOM they're

pregnant.

This is what happened to me when I was trying to get my hair back. I was so focused on my hair growing in that I was scared to take a shower, I was constantly running to the mirror to see any sign of hair regrowth! Finally, I just had an epiphany. That day I took a shower I vowed to stop stressing and to trust the process of healing. More importantly, I had to trust myself. I stopped worrying and stressing every frigging second of my life and actually allow the change to affect me. It's not just about letting go of, It's about making room for…I had to keep moving forward and have fun with it.

Mental stagnation will throw you off from reaching your goal. Just know that if you are truly doing this healthy philosophy, your body will reward you. There will be no more reasons to worry. Health is your bodies answer, regardless of what the back of poisonous medicine bottles promise. Toxicity will always come with a backlash (if not now, than later) that will eventually hit you right in the ass. Organic Fruits and Vegetables are nature's true medicine full of nutrient rich vitamins, minerals, anti-oxidants, fiber, calcium, potassium, plenty of vitamin C (and other nutrients).

Those are the human species true universal healers. Fresh produce does not come with warning labels, disclaimers or "keep out of reach of children & pregnant women" risks. What we take in is our only REAL solution! Not some fake, profitable B.S.

The only one who will be reaping rewards is yourself, or the people you will naturally inspire while living this naturally delicious, healing lifestyle. Enjoy experiencing freedom.

Yoga

My mom met a woman at the chiropractor's office, whom she started to go to health workshops with. Gladis is an older woman and anyone's inspiration for how to live a healthy lifestyle. She asked my mom to go to a yoga class, insisting Mom would love it. After some time of Gladis persistently asking and raving about yoga, my mom gave in and went. Little did she know that Bikram yoga takes place in an uncomfortably heated room. She was wearing pants and a long-sleeved shirt, and nearly fell to the floor, lying in a pool of sweat. She didn't go back to Bikram yoga, but she did love the whole idea of yoga. She ended up going to a regular yoga class practiced in a nice room in someone's huge beach front home. When she came back from her first class, she was calm. And she started begging me to go. I was about thirteen and a half years old.

After a while I agreed to go, but only because she bribed me, telling me how nice the house was. I love architecture. I also love getting up early in the morning and taking a nice country drive. I wore a hat with my hairpiece underneath, so that when I did any head-down poses, my hair would stay on. Plus, I always wore my hairpiece around new people.

This class didn't go that well for me. It wasn't that I didn't like yoga, I just couldn't concentrate and get into the "serenity" feelings with my hairpiece falling forward every time I bent down. I was saving my dignity by not putting my head all the way down when I did a bend. It was awkward, not being able to go into some of the poses appropriately. My tense, inflexible muscles didn't help.

Other than that I loved the people there and gobbled up the attention of being the only child in the class, so I kept going with my mom. After a while we became so friendly with all of the people there, Mom told them about my alopecia. I didn't mind. Once I learned I could trust all of them, they encouraged me to take off my hairpiece. I was annoyed with not being able to do yoga properly and not experiencing the great feeling I was supposed to have, so one day I decided to leave the wig behind. I was nervous as hell about their reaction, but everyone was unbelievably kind and welcoming. It was a huge relief not to have a ponytail in my face anymore.

My experience with yoga after that was everything my mom had said it would be. Serenity was an understatement of how great I felt. Even though my poses were a little tight, I had become more flexible. The owner of the yoga studio, Casey, is a true yogi with a passion for her practice. She said to me, "The pain you feel as you first go into a position that's tight is a sensation." I thought she was a little crazy. There was no way the feeling I was getting came close to a "sensation." It was more like "intolerable." But there was something addictive about the feeling of contentment and happiness after yoga that I couldn't resist. I needed that light feeling more than anything at that time. After practicing the positions, I was able to let go of my tense muscles, once I learned to let go of the tensions I was feeling in general. It was mind over matter. I just had to keep practicing until that intolerable feeling went away and was completely replaced by the sensational feeling Casey was talking about. That's when I started feeling the true benefits of yoga. By letting go, my muscles were able to relax and I could mentally guide my breath throughout my body, so the clean air washed away toxicities as rain does for the earth. This is important for the release of not just toxins in the body, but toxins in the mind as well. I never felt so good. In fact, I felt like I was "walking on sunshine."

I started to use a yoga DVD at home, so I could really enjoy it. I did it in the living room at first, but that didn't work. Between my father and brother getting up to go to work, my mom walking by, the dogs licking my face, and my cat seducing me by circling my body, purring, I kept getting distracted. Where else could I go? I wasn't going to let a couple of intrusions take me away from my yoga practice, so I went into the basement and found a small TV. I threw a DVD player on it and squeezed my yoga mat in between my treadmill and the ironing board. At the time I didn't have a yoga strap (To use if you can't reach your hands to your feet or because you're not flexible enough), so I used a leather belt. For a yoga block I used my shoe. Determination is an understatement for me. Nothing stands in my way when it comes to routines that I feel are important. The appearance of where I was practicing yoga did not detract from the importance of the practice. Somehow I found serenity and peace. Instead of complaining about the ugly, dark gray environment, I told myself it was a peaceful surrounding. That I felt grounded being so near to the ground. That's not me convincing myself; that's me motivating myself. I was seeking truth in positive words instead of complaining and subconsciously psyching myself out, so that I would neglect something so important.

Now I could feel why it was so vital to go into the positions fully and put my head completely down when I needed to. Doing a downward dog, pushing my hands into the floor and encouraging my heels to touch the ground, I released all of the tension in the back of my neck, my shoulders, and the muscles of my torso, giving the tension to my legs. Then the tension vanished as I breathed. I quieted my mind, which was much needed. The calm of yoga comes from every stretch, as you release toxins throughout your body and eliminate them through your breath. Your mind is so quiet, just watching what pose you go into, breathing in, and then breathing out through the pose. I strongly believe yoga is something you simply have to do in a busy world full of to-do lists. Just stop, stretch, and breathe. It's easier for me to stay positive when I'm relaxed and have my head on straight, making my thoughts clear and my mind present. Yoga took away that emotionally draining pain inside my chest.

When I miss a yoga practice or forget even to take a couple of yoga breaths, close my eyes, and realize where I am and how much I got myself through, I again feel those haunted emotions I used to have. Yoga forces me to let go and give up my pain. It helps me stay grounded and present. Every pose makes me more and more aware of where I am. With every practice I keep feeling lighter and lighter.

In yoga, each pose squeezes different internal organs, helping to release toxins. I didn't realize that because I was so tense, I didn't go to the bathroom often enough. If that's not harmful to my body, then I don't know what is! Yoga reduced my anxiety and tension; I could actually feel them fading away. That gave my body the opportunity to focus on healing my immune system.

I also realized that it really made a difference being around the positive people at the yoga studio. They got me out of my shell, and I actually came alive.

I have developed a few other quick fixes for my mindset, when it's not practical to do a full yoga routine. The trick is to do anything that allows you to be present and to focus on what's important. Sometimes I get so caught up in my problems, I forget what's going on around me. Whenever I can't get out of my head and my decisions don't make sense, I know it's to go lie down or take a nap. Other times, when I just need a brief break, I sit on my front steps and become present and aware. My mind stops and I focus my thought on the sounds of nature. My favorite sound in the world is birds communicating.

I also like to go for walks, with or without our dogs. When I'm around our pets, I frequently stop and pet them, allowing myself to be as present as they are.

My mom and I love soundtracks from favorite movies. Listening to them always puts a smile on my face, especially the soundtrack from *Under the Tuscan Sun*, staring Diane Lane. In the movie, the main character goes through a terrible time and ends up making a new and better life for herself. I can relate. Whenever I listen to that soundtrack, I feel empowered.

I also listen to comedy CDs. They're a great way to enhance my thoughts and just laugh. I hadn't laughed so long as I did when I listened to Dane Cook's comedy CD. I laughed so hard I was crying, and it glued a smile on my face for a long time. It gave my mind some relief and my body felt better than ever.

My family has also found that one way to be truly positive is to keep positive people in our lives. It's amazing how, when we only associate with people who actually enjoy life, how much more we smile. This is a huge key in the elimination process. I had to learn how to filer out all the negative people in my life in order to become a mindful, positive person. My family and I plucked out all the people who had a negative impact on us and could affect us in a poor way. People influence people. I noticed my thoughts were more positive without Mr. Melancholy and Ms. Sarcastic bringing me down. The result for all of us was a much lighter and less tense household.

Inspirational Audio Books

An audio book that both my mom and I love is called *The Last Lecture*. It's about a professor of computer science named Randy Pausch. When he was forty-five he was diagnosed with terminal pancreatic cancer and wrote a book about his last lecture, which he gave less than a year before he died. That last lecture revolved around the question, "What wisdom would you try to impart to the world if it was your last chance?" His answer—really achieving your childhood dreams.

The question is a typical one, but not in his situation. Just listening to him opened my eyes. It was moving to hear how strong he was. The way he went about the most "terminal" time of his life taught me so much.

Books are, of course, a great source of information, and audio books are a terrific way to be inspired and motivated. One of my all-time favorite audio books is *The China Study*. After listening to this, let's just say I never have a tough time ordering healthy food when I got out to eat. The authors, T. Colin Campbell, PhD, and his son, Thomas M. Campbell, MD, will blow your mind with information that you should know about what you're eating. Even my brother put down his sports magazine to listen and ask questions. This book is informative, helpful, and will be eye-opening for you and your family. It gave me another direction to guide me on my health path.

Those are my favorite books, which were really life changing for me and opened my eyes to see past a disease. I recognized the power of thought, and how my thinking cannot just create my daily routines, but make them staples in my life that I actually went to get up and do.

Sleep

My lifestyle is full of essential routines that require stability. Sleep is one of them. If I don't get the right amount of sleep, I'm a wreck like most people. All routines require discipline. If I can't discipline myself to go to bed at a time that allows me to get eight to ten hours of sleep, then how am I going to live a balanced life when I'm not a balanced human being? If I couldn't convince myself to maintain a discipline routine that ensures balance, then I wasn't in the proper mindset even to get out of bed or turn off the TV. Let alone make healthy food and exercise. I became aware that when I was tired, I didn't do things correctly. It is best for me to catch up for an hour or so immediately, instead of paying for it for the next few days. Being susceptible to disease, my body needs sleep in order to heal and recover. The body goes into restoration mode when it's snoozing (hence the names beauty sleep and rest and repair). If it's asking for sleep, I have learned to take the hint, let go, and nap. This is especially important for my overall energy and awareness. I know if I don't get my sleep, I feel light-headed and unconsciously distort my whole routine.

This goes for friends as well. If you have that one person in your life (Late-night Lucy or Party Peter) who insists you stay up with them or go out late at night, think about yourself. If that's going to interfere with your sleep routine, don't go.

My family and I are huge advocates on the importance of sleep and how cat naps can help you stay refreshed, aware, and have an overall great day. I never let fatigue own me. I eliminate it by going into my room, shutting the shades, and taking a nap. If I'm not home when tiredness hits, I get in my car, lock the doors, and recline my seat all the way back. I take a nap or just rest my eyes to gain more awareness. Doing this helps me feel grounded and clear headed, so I can keep up with my everyday life while enjoying it. When your body asks for sleep, it's important to listen. Sleep restores the body, and now that I get as much as I need, the quality of my life has completely shifted. It's as if I had blurred vision and now can see clearly. I've heard people say they only get four or five hours of sleep a night and it's all they need. But that's only because they've gotten used to that short snooze pattern. The body can go on like for only so long like that (like a windup doll, it suddenly will stop working).

Movement

"Those who think they have no time for bodily exercise will soon or later have to find time for illness." - Edward Stanley

Although I consider yoga exercise and as necessary for the body as the mind, I believe just as much in the power of more traditional exercise. Cardiovascular exercise and strength training help the body naturally detoxify itself, working hand and hand with a healthy diet. Sweating through your pores, especially during a cardio routine, has a cleansing and detoxifying effect. Toxins are being released from the inside out. My workout routine is simple. I joined a gym, where I walk or jog on the treadmill, do some strength training with light weights, and focus on yoga. Also I leave myself with enough energy to play basketball or ride my bike. As long as I'm moving my body and not sitting every second, that's all that matters. It completes my lifestyle of healthy living.

There are all different forms of exercise. Sometimes I get sick of the same boring routine and don't want to go to the gym. I've learned that it's okay not to go to the gym every day, just as long as I move my body in some fashion. The same thing happens, no matter how I exercise. When I don't go to the gym, I make sure I do something—shoot hoops, hike, walk, swim, run, walk the mall, or yoga. There are so many ways to move my body! My routine is not boring, and that way it's realistic. I take bits and pieces of different exercises and forms of movement and incorporate them into my schedule. I don't have to go to boot camp to stay in shape and be healthy. That wouldn't last very long anyway. I just get my body moving.

Movement is beyond being skinny and looking good. When my body is in motion, I notice I feel happier. That's my brain releasing healthy chemicals called endorphins. Endorphins reduce the perception of pain, which makes for a natural alternative to medication. Also, exercise reduces my stress, making me feel more positive and enlightened, with an energizing outlook on life.

Regular exercise has proven to: reduce stress, ward off anxiety and depression, boost self-esteem, and improve sleep. On top of all that it also: strengthens your heart; increases energy levels; lowers blood pressure; improves muscle tone and strength; strengthens and builds bones; helps reduce fat, which is toxic and a burden to the body; and keeps your body fit and healthy from the inside out. Exercise is an effective yet underused and underestimated treatment for some health problems. Most people can only look at exercise as a way of enhancing their appearance, but in fact exercise has natural healing abilities and should be given more credit for that.

Diet

"High-tech tomatoes. Mysterious milk. Supersquash. Are we supposed to eat this stuff? Or is it going to eat us?" - Annita Manning

Being homeschooled, I had a lot of time to think. I had the luxury of independently studying on my own. I started to research more about alopecia on the Internet. Still no luck learning anything new. I didn't give up researching, though. I did read about the chemicals that are in household cleaners, lawn pesticides, and other everyday household items. I read that they can be harmful to our bodies. I had my mom come in and read what I was studying. That day we went out and stocked out shelves with nontoxic cleaners.

This really intrigued me, and I kept studying chemicals, poisons, and toxins that we come into contact with in our everyday lives. That's when I found organic food and learned that whatever food I ate that was not certified as organic had chemicals. I was eating chemicals? I told that to my mom, and she said she had heard of organic food but had never looked into it. She read what I had found and was disgusted. She was making chicken for dinner that night, and with what we had just learned, we couldn't eat it. Not when we knew that a nonorganic chicken was pumped with poisonous chemical and fed a poor diet to fatten it up.

When I picture a farm where chickens are raised for our consumption, I picture green grass and a barnyard filled with free range birds, white picket fences, and a couple of clean chicken coops. My picture is correct, but that's how a farm that raises chickens organically looks. A conventional, nonorganic farm resembles overheated housing in which chicken are all stuffed in the same place, living and dead chickens in there together. The chickens are injected with steroids to pump up their muscle tone like body builders, so that they can feed the ever-growing human population. All those steroids end up inside the person who choose to eat that chicken. A little different than an organically raised chicken, I would say. This goes for all animal foods, except for seafood. Seafood is best when it's wild. Wild fish are usually healthier (high in omega-3) and less contaminated than farm-raised fish.

So I eat the organic food, saving myself from poison in all foods. That chicken was the start of it for me. I got back to the basics—you are what you eat.

"The better the quality of food you consume the less chemically-induced damage your body will have to repair."

(Wellnessresources.com)

***

When I lost my hair, I tried figuring how it happened. It's like when you break up with someone. You keep wondering, *What happened? What could I have done differently?* These questions about alopecia were always front and center in my mind. I kept trying to find a reason for how it had happened, or "why me?" When I researched and found information on toxicity in the body and healthy organic foods, I started thinking outside the box a bit more. Since I couldn't answer any of the questions in my head and find anything I could have done differently, I thought about the food I had eaten my whole life. My family were average Americans eating a typical toxic-food diet. I didn't realize until then the impact my diet had on my body. If eating organic foods meant I wouldn't be eating foods that were sprayed with poison, then what was my family eating? It's like your favorite fast-food restaurant chain announcing that it is now serving "white" meat. Well, what was it serving before? I realized I might be onto something here. Maybe it was a piece of my mom's intuitive feeling.

I couldn't come up with an answer for *why me?* But if I couldn't find a reason for why this has happened to me, then maybe I should stop asking myself questions and go more into the present here. In reality I had alopecia and not a clue why. In reality I was eating poisoned food. So, in order to be present and stop thinking about pointless questions, my new goal was to eat organic foods and think about the ingredients I should be eating. I wanted to fuel my body with clean nutrients and heal it from poisoned foods. I wasn't sure there was a connection between eating toxic food and losing my hair. What I did know was that although I did not have control over my alopecia, I did have control over what foods I put into my body. Food was a decision I could make every day that could affect my body in a positive way and help it heal or maintain good health. Food could also affect my body negatively. It was obvious to me that chemically-enhanced foods could hurt my body. That was the last thing a person with an autoimmune disease needed.

My mom and I agreed that I should remove refined carbohydrates, refined sugars, gluten, and red meat from my diet. I suspected they could increase a person's susceptibility to autoimmune diseases since they all strain digestion, keep toxicity inside, and are refined. When a food is refined, it means the only nutritious part of the food has been taken out by processing, which is why refined foods are also called processed foods. There is nothing good for you when it comes to foods that have no nutritional value! I started to eat more vegetables, fruit, nuts, seeds, whole grains, fish, and poultry. This diet aided my digestion and helped naturally detox my body frequently, instead of sporadically. Red meat, gluten, refined carbs, and refined sugars bog my body down. Those foods are hard to digest, so they can just sit in the colon and ferment. Now that's toxic!

The first thing my mom and I noticed was that the price of organic food was higher than conventional food. We figured, though, we pay now or we pay later. My family made the choice to put our money into our health, which is the best investment. Our dollars go to the food we consume and not to visits to the doctor's office and to medicines. I would like to point out that we rarely get sick anymore.

At that time my dad purchased four or five cups of coffee every day from his favorite coffee shop chain. We broke down the cost of that small yet unhealthy habit. He was paying $3770 a year for false energy! He was happy to stop drinking his cups of Joe. First he drank only one or two cups of organic coffee at home. Then he weaned himself off coffee entirely, drinking decaffeinated herbal tea and a green smoothie once a day that he made at home. He understood that organic food was more important than his unhealthy habit. We chose the obvious— healthy instead of unhealthy.

From a young age I had always looked forward to mealtime and appreciated good food. It was normal in my house to order pizza and subs a couple of nights a week for dinner. Other nights we had comfort foods—meat, potatoes, and a vegetable. During the day I usually ate quick foods, especially sandwiches, which I enjoyed making. The first time my mom allowed me to use the kitchen on my own, I made a cold-cut sandwich.

Of course, we also loved going to your average fast-food restaurant. I'd order the norm: chicken fingers and fries with a soda, and if I was feeling jazzy, a vanilla sundae too. Not to mention that my family also went out to dinner at least once a week to the same handful of restaurants that we considered "the best." Since we frequented the same restaurants, my parents had made friends with the people that worked there. My brother and I used to order off the kid's menu, until my parents encouraged us to keep trying their meals. Our tastes quickly changed. We went from eating chicken fingers and fries to chicken Parmesan. We were practically professional orderers. The friends we had at the time were always ordering pizza and kid food, and we would say, "No, try this." We love great-tasting food so much that we also loved cooking at home. I remember that once my palate was accustomed to such flavors, I didn't want to eat anything other than rich, delicious foods. I guess you could say I have a spoiled palate. Honestly, if it doesn't taste good, it's not worth eating. Every restaurant we ate at, I ate like a queen. It's hard to top food so rich—and by rich, I mean foods pretty much drowning in buttery sauces. The average meal was not good enough for my brother and I. My parents probably wondered what monsters they'd created, but they were just as wild for this food. Every meal had to be a taste explosion or our senses would be bored. My mom had a hard time keeping up with our new preferences, but since we were homeschooled, we went out to lunch a lot. Eating healthy wasn't on our minds at the time, but when I made it my goal to be healthy, it definitely was anything but easy. We stocked out kitchen with all organic food, but we didn't really know what to do with it. Organic food tastes cleaner than its chemically infused alternative, but that does not mean it has to be plain. We were letting our thoughts about something we considered foreign make this so much more complicated than it had to be. My mom started to cook out of cookbooks. If the ingredients called for milk, she would use organic coconut or rice milk. If it called for butter, she replaced it with organic ghee (clarified butter) or regular organic butter, but she would use a quarter of the amount. My brother and I, being the food critics that we are, would tentatively take a first bite, scared it would taste like monkey poop, but our expectations were always wrong. Now that we were cooking with fresh organic foods, everything had such a clear, light, and rich taste to it. Before, I had thought happiness was at the bottom of a cookie box. Now happiness derives from how good I feel and how much energy I have.

I avoided buying any unhealthy foods. I figured if I wanted to avoid them, then don't buy them? That was my way of moving forward and trying to make progress. I had to let my body puts its energy into the right places, allowing it to heal itself. Especially since my body was combating a disease. How could my body be focused on healing itself when it was trying to figure out what the hell I was eating and what it had to assimilate?

Just because I had stumbled across organic food and was now on the health track, did not mean I stopped learning. As I kept researching, I found quite a few articles and websites about the green smoothie. It was touted as the best thing you can do for your health. Since this was nutrition in a cup, it aided my digestion like nobody's business. That helped me naturally detox and purify my body while the nutrients brushed my intestinal track. The intestines are twenty feet long! Imagine if all that is full of old food, caught in the creases of the colon. When I discuss smoothies I don't mean to add in powered products just simple water, fruit and mostly vegetables. Trust me, it's delicious!

Most people are used to getting their energy from caffeinated drinks. How about a smoothie instead? I promise your body will not crash later. Smoothies give your body natural (real!) energy by feeding your whole body, not just triggering your brain like a wind-up doll.

My family and I started making smoothies with a regular kitchen blender. We ended up burning out the motor on that thing with a few experiments. My mom decided to buy a commercial grade blender. She chose a Vitamix. It was a little pricey, but five years later it's still running like new. And the smooth texture it brought to the smoothies was priceless.

Initially I made my smoothies with water, various fruits, leafy greens, and other vegetables. Just enough for a twenty-ounce smoothie. Then I started to have fun with smoothie making to keep my taste buds and senses alive and not bored with the same drink every day. To the fruit, greens, and veggies I added different ingredients, like vanilla, coconut milk, cinnamon, almond butter, hemp butter, and even pumpkin pie spice. I just kept it healthy. I'm so good at making great-tasting smoothies, they taste like a frappe or my favorite ice cream. But when I go to bed at night, I actually think about how I want morning to come so I can have what I call my treat! The amount of produce that are in my smoothies is more than I used to consume in a week. Now I'm downing it and enjoying it every day. (At the back of the book, I've added the recipes for some of my favorite smoothies, as well as other recipes.)

If you choose to eat organic, be sure the food you are buying is truly organic. Make certain it has a label that says "Certified Organic." This means that the government certified the farm(s) are up to the standards approved by the United States Department of Agriculture (USDA). To reap the benefits of organic food while not emptying your bank account, The Environmental Working Group (www.foodnews.org) has validated that certain produce are treated with far less pesticides. All the produce on "The Clean 15" bore little to no traces of pesticides, and is safe to consume in non-organic form. This list includes:

- onions
- avocados
- sweet corn
- pineapples
- mango

- sweet peas
- asparagus
- kiwi fruit
- cabbage
- eggplant
- cantaloupe
- watermelon
- grapefruit
- sweet potatoes"

Eating healthy is just about simplicity. Only yous make it complicated. What I do everyday is going what my body is going to build off of. So I'd choose a fresh organic apple that contains living nutrients instead of a processed cookie that I'll eat every now and then.

The foods we eat consistently are always organic. Remember that you are what you do, and what you eat. I can't say that enough.

Sometimes it just takes persistence and consistency to break down your walls that keep you from all things different. I always gave myself credit and supported myself through these sometimes difficult transitions.

Detox

Since I was eating so clean and healthy, naturally enhancing my digestive system and promoting healthy bowel movements, my body went into detox mode. I hadn't realized how much old food (feces) was weighing my body down. When old food sits too long in the body, it ferments, just as you think anything that expires would. That promotes illness and disease. Everybody's body speaks to them different, and our change in diet had a different effect on my mom. For years she had had to take medication for high cholesterol. She also had suffered with irritable bowel syndrome (IBS). I remember her in a cold sweat, sprawled out on the bathroom floor like wet paint.

Who knew eating healthy food would affect every single aspect of our lives? My whole family's life changed, and my mom's IBS vanished unbelievably quickly. We don't feel like walking trash cans anymore holding in smelly garbage. Think of what that was doing to our health. In my experience, poor eating habits lead to sickness and disease.

***

I kept reading, and for the first time I truly knew I was on the right path, just as my mom's instincts had told her. Detox is the body ridding itself of toxins that are poisonous to the system. *Bingo.* Right there I knew I was on the right track. My body had to start over.

The way I pictured detox was by thinking of a baby. Babies are in their purest form when they are born. They are (mostly) clean, clear vessels with a pure body, flawless skin, clear eyes, and clean thoughts. They are the perfect human being. Detox would allow me to begin again. I could rid myself of all the toxins that could be hurting my body. Since diseases and illnesses take place inside the body, I directed my mind to the source.

As a busy participant in everyday life, consumed by my habits and schedule, when I first developed alopecia I knew nothing about how my body worked. If you had asked me when I was twelve, I would have probably brought up the food pyramid that I was taught in "health" class in my old school by an overweight teacher. If he said anything about body mechanics, it flew right over my head.

Just like everyone else I knew, I patronized the subject of health by eating a side of vegetables that had been microwaved in a plastic bag. Truth is, if you don't know how important health is, then you just don't know. If my dad was taught by his father that franks and beans are good food, then franks and beans are what's for dinner. Odds are he will eat that way until he learns differently. Once he learns, it's up to him to change his eating habits. Or not.

You are learning information about health from me right now. In the end, though, these are just words on paper. Although these words are true and hopefully inspiring does not mean you are actually going to pursue this health process. You might even try this lifestyle and then eat that piece of pie you were trying to resist and realize you just don't have the will power to undertake such a big change. Or if you are older and have lived with alopecia for many years, you might tell yourself that you're too old even to consider switching your lifestyle. Or if you're a child like I was, you're probably in a hurry to get your hair back, so you'll try anything.

This book is meant for all people of all ages, to inspire and motivate. This book is meant to address something bigger than a disease. This book is about health. Your one body is for some reason fighting with itself. This lifestyle can reset that defensive mode. Don't look at these suggestions as obstacles, but as parts of a fun transition for yourself. I got excited about my life switch as I established my new lifestyle and watched my body eliminate toxins and evolve into radiant health. I feel reborn, with no inner flaws. Isn't that how everyone should feel?

After I felt so good from eliminating all toxins from my home and body, I came to the point of automatic health. I felt amazing, and that's the key to knowing I had evolved into a state of consistent healing. I knew I could always remain healed if I kept my life clean and toxin free. I loved my new life, and the irony is, if I hadn't had alopecia, I would never have found wellness. Being susceptible to a disease is like living with a strict coach with a piercing whistle, who's trying to keep me on track for my own good.

***

You may be a beginner in the learning stages of healthy living, but so what? I didn't know everything about how to be healthy. I started with pieces of information I happened to find while doing research. But at least I got off my chair and got moving once I was educated. I would've killed for a book like this that laid out the path for me, that showed me that someone was out there who had my condition and was in full control of it. You have this book. Start with the information I have provided and build off what you know. Sometimes we know the right thing to do by instinct, common sense, or just connecting some dots of information that we've gathered from other people and our experiences. This process that I am advocating is not a treatment. It is a lifestyle, and it is completely in your hands.

Your own great health is your journey, not a destination. You are the vehicle that will undergo this journey. All you have to do is make the decision to drive.

If you ask me, good health is more promising than steroid shots and just makes more sense as a whole. Treatments are a way to "cheat the system" by trying to put a patch on what's wrong. I chose to revive myself with health. I could have easily stayed bald and tried steroid shots, which would have poisoned not just my head, but my whole body. If I went that direction, guess where I would be? Bald and scheduling steroid shots, hoping they would work. Instead I chose what I think was the harder route, but more rewarding in the long run. I took the time and made changes that resulted in a different lifestyle, not a schedule. Yes, it took work to gain first the knowledge and then the health, but I did it. While some people are heading to the doctors' for their next painful injection, I'm at home getting ready to work out and preparing a healthy meal.

***

Growing up, I thought heavy people were just heavy and skinny people were skinny. I also thought that if you got a clean bill of health from the doctor after your yearly physical, then you were healthy and free of disease. It's not that simple. You become what you eat over time. Whether you become overweight, have digestive issues, or something more serious such as heart disease of type 2 diabetes, an effect is an effect and always has a cause. Most body issues are overthought. So many people are looking for the answer or the cure and ignoring what they eat every day.

Feed your body what it wants and then see what happens.

For the first time I had to feed my body and not my cravings. I had to think about what I *should* be eating, not what I *wanted* to eat. That's not an easy task for anyone, but I stopped making it a task and made it a lifestyle choice. I made it a routine to get up every morning, make a smoothie, and make sure I have healthy snacks to eat throughout the day. I wasn't being forced to do this; it all came down to what I wanted. I had to push past my comfort zone in order to get it, but now I'm proud of the way I eat and the choices I make. As my friends are ordering greasy pizzas and eating candy bars, I made my own pizzas with fresh

ingredients and my much healthier desserts. I enjoy my

decisions for myself because they make me feel good. I respect

health, and I do put my own great health on a pedestal. My new

life decisions flipped my worst days of worrying about my hair

to results I once could have only dreamed of.

Once I stopped overthinking my health and stopped looking at it

like a science experiment, everything fell into place. Naturally.

What is so great about routines is that you become what you do

repeatedly.

Vitamins

During my journey of researching, I learned that vitamins are crucial for health and are usually what a lot of people lack. Common sense told me not just to take any candy-flavored vitamin in the shape of a cute animal, but *essential* vitamins. Since I felt so good with my new lifestyle, why not add something that's so essential for my health? So I started to take:

Fish oil—1-2 teaspoons of the liquid form or 4 capsules. Most people complain about the taste of the liquid form, but when it's lemon flavored, it tastes like an oily lemon. Which is nothing to complain about, especially when my body needs it. Fish oil contains important omega-3s. According to cleanseyourbody.com, fish oil can help lubricate joints, prevent heart disease, aid in cancer treatment, and help protect the brain from Alzheimer disease. Not to mention that fish oil also help my digestion with its anti-inflammatory properties in the intestines and tissues.

Probiotics are the bacteria that exist in the gastrointestinal track and which support digestion and the immune system. I consider probiotics important for healthy digestion.

Vitamin D is vital for proper immune system functioning, bone development, and calcium absorption. It helps maintain healthy muscle mass, especially for someone who exercises a lot. Life tends to take over, and sometimes it's just not possible to get twenty minutes of sunlight a day. Vitamin D capsules ensure that I give my body the vitamin it needs.

These essential vitamins are, well, essential. Important!

Crucial! These are nutrients that the body simply needs more of

most of the time, and vitamins fill that gap of vital nutrients we

often lack.

Water, Water, Water!

We all know we need water, one of the essential

elements on earth, to stay alive. We need water like we need

food and air. I used to have little symptoms that had everything

to do with dehydration, I just didn't know it at the time. I had no

idea I was supposed to be drinking at least sixty-four ounces a

day! Honestly, I think I drank eight ounces (one cup) a day, if

that. In the morning I would have a glass of orange juice, which

was anything but freshly squeezed. It was more like drinking

candy. Throughout the day I would have soda, more sugary

juice, and sports drinks. I never drank water! Once I was

educated and actually started to drink more water, my body felt

as clean as the water.

We are a water-based life-form; our bodies are 60-70 percent

water. I started to gulp water in the morning and noticed I felt different. Not just awake, but wide awake. I thought about how long I slept—approximately ten hours. It wasn't like I drank while sleeping, so my body went that long without water. In the morning I'm obviously going to have to step up my water intake, drinking more then and then gradually less throughout the day. I might urinate more frequently, but that's the way the body purifies itself. When I started to drink more water, I noticed that not just my morning fatigue went away, but I wasn't as tired throughout the day.

I have common allergies, and staying hydrated helped with those. Also, I can think clearly without forgetting or getting random headaches. Not only have my allergies, headaches, and fatigue stopped, but my skin has been extra clear as well.

Since our bodies work on water to keep us ticking, a couple of glasses a day are not going to do the job of making sure the whole body is getting properly hydrated. My family buys packs of twenty-four water bottles to keep in each car, so when we're not at home, we have no excuse not to stay hydrated. Who needs energy drinks? Not me! My energy is linked to how hydrated I am, on top of my lifestyle as a whole. My inner body doesn't resemble a desert anymore. Please, don't forget to recycle your bottles.

Food also plays a big role in hydrating the body. Raw vegetables, leafy greens, and fruit all contain a huge amount of water. That's why smoothies and salads are so vital for health. What happens to your body when you're dehydrated?

Your brain won't work properly. You'll be groggy, slow, and feel out of it.

You'll lose muscle tone.

Your kidneys won't be able to function.

You'll have trouble regulating your body temperature.

You may feel overheated, or you may feel chronically

106

cold.

You'll get constipated.

Fats stored in your body won't get used up or metabolized.

You'll think you're hungry all the time, so you'll be likely to eat more.

Your skin will get dry, itchy, and saggy.

Putting it all together

A year and a half after I started changing my lifestyle, my hair began growing back in patchy spots. My mom told me I was beating the odds, even though doctors had told me I would never see a strand of hair again. I grabbed onto what my mom said and told myself how lucky I was to have any hair, even if it was short and sparse. I was pretty enough, and short hair brought out my big blue eyes.

As the hair stayed, I got more confident that I could grow hair. I got it through my head (literally) that I *was* beating the odds. I kept my hairpiece off as much as possible, figuring I should let my real hair breathe, since my head had been suffocating all these years.

My head hadn't gotten any sunlight for quite some time, or my body, so I started to play outside in the sun and lie on a lawn chair in my driveway. I would uncover my bald spots, let the sun hit them for twenty minutes, and encourage my body to let the light sink in and absorb the nutrients I'd lacked for so long. I also got a nice tan and stopped resembling Caspar the Ghost from always hiding in my house or under a hat. As I let my head breathe and got more comfortable with taking my hairpiece off more often, my mom and I wondered why my hair wasn't growing in fully.

I was happy to be growing hair at all—it had been so long since I'd lost my hair, I'd forgotten I could even grow it—but I was still disturbed that I didn't have *all* of my hair. Why bald spots? My scattered hair matched my scattered thoughts. My mom's thoughts, on the other hand, were more realistic. She told me to remember that my body was still trying to recover. I had replaced my bad habits—poor diet, negative mindset, lack of exercise—and now I had to let my body do its job. I had to keep going with my routine at a steady pace that could last my whole life. Healing wasn't going to be a case of a swing of the wand and, *poof*, I had my hair back. It was a process that my body had to go through.

To keep my mindset positive, I did not run to the mirror every morning to see if more hair was filling in. Instead, I kept picturing myself at my healthiest with no toxicity. Yes, that thought included an image of me with a full head of hair and glowing skin. I pictured myself not just with hair like I used to have, but as a radiantly healthy human being. As long as I had that mental picture on top of my daily healthy routines, I remained confident that the best life waited for me.

Alopecia Areata & Totalis

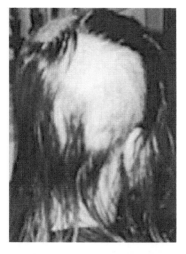

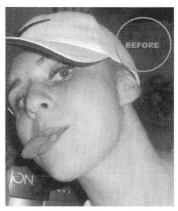

Which quickly started to turn into

Alopecia Universalis (all body hair gone).

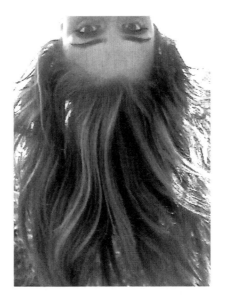

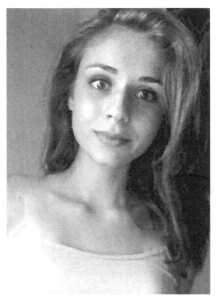

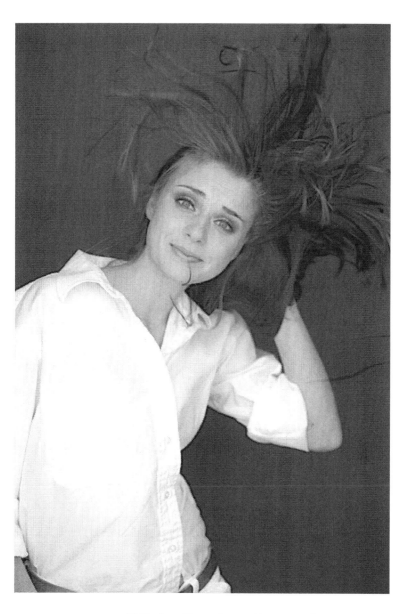

This Is the Result

When my hair started growing back, I didn't feel the way I had expected. I thought I would jump for joy or be so wide-eyed, that I couldn't sleep. Instead, I felt humbled. I felt comfort, warmth, and security, as if I had watched a dying tree come to life again, sprouting leaves and blossoms. My mind had reached a state of ease, my life a love of joy, and I couldn't have asked for anything more. I just laid my emotions to rest.

Since doctors had said my hair loss was permanent, I was afraid my hair would fall out again. I didn't want to descend to that level of disappointment once more, so I focused on the hair that I had and not the scared emotions that followed. That effort was simple, because I had learned to let go of what was going on with my hair. I embraced life and all the positive things that were blossoming in it. I just remained grateful for the fact that I was on the path of wellness and my hair was growing in because of my lifestyle choices.

When my hair reached the length I called boy-short, I embraced the new look and started to dress in more girly clothes. At that point I couldn't help feeling excited about having hair again. I balanced my anxiety about losing my hair again with my joyful emotions. My wardrobe went from dark, sad colors (black, navy, gray) to happy colors (pink, lime green, sky blue, orange, and white). I dressed how I felt! As I changed my wardrobe, I gained more energy from all the happy endorphins running through my body. I sang my lungs out when music was on. That was my way of celebrating what I'd accomplished.

A year went by, and by the time I was fifteen my hair was down to my shoulders. My family took a vacation that year to Disney World. It was our first vacation since my hair had started growing back, and it was my favorite trip ever. My brother and I ran around like we were little kids again, and my parents glowed with delight to see their daughter happy again. Because I was happy and felt free, my whole family felt the same way. We were all shining free spirits having the best time of our lives, celebrating my new happiness and the positive, healthy life we were all embracing.

***

All of the knowledge I gleaned in my research would have been useless if I hadn't made the first move to incorporate it into my life. I had to take action. As I let go and trusted that I was on the right path of health, everything fell into place. But the hardest part of getting on a healthy track was finding foods I actually liked. I've had my fair share of granola that tasted like sawdust, of trying tofu and gagging at its spongy consistency and bland taste, of buying whole-wheat pizzas that were as soft as shoe leather. I did notice that the fewer ingredients in prepackaged food, the better the food tasted. Eventually I found new staple foods that I loved.

I really like going to the grocery store now. It's an adventure on its own, searching for the simplest ingredients. Just knowing a food is healthy and tastes really good makes it fun. I pick out snacks like seed crackers, baked corn chips, salsa, and chocolate chip cookies made from whole grain flours. Yum.

I don't subsist on bland foods just because they're considered healthy. If something doesn't taste good, I find a way to make it better. There is nothing worse than being ready to eat your lunch and it's disgusting, but you feel you have to eat it because it's healthy. Not in my kitchen. I may have started that way, but once I got the hang of foods that are simple, healthy, and taste good, sayonara bland foods that taste like a foot and hello mouth-watering dishes I look forward to eating.

Looking back on the way I used to eat makes me sick. I honestly can't believe I ate like that. My brother comes home from work and tells me what his work buddy ate that day: processed cakes wrapped in cellophane, a bag of cheese-sprayed fried chips, and a green soda to wash it all down. I tell him I'm thankful I know about the importance of eating healthy, because if you don't know, then you just don't know. Sometimes, as in my case, it takes an illness to bring the importance of health into your life. Seeing the way we live now, you would never know my mom made microwaved cheese-covered broccoli only a few years ago. We replaced the microwave with a toaster oven to avoid cooking with radiation that ends up in our foods. It's not that hard to reheat leftovers in a pan on the stovetop.

That was my normal, my family's normal, and most of America's normal. But there is nothing normal about that way of eating. And it's not only what we eat, but also how much we eat. I was brought up to eat that way, however, and I knew no different than the people around me. I learned and watched my parents eat this food, and was fed this food as a child, just as my parents were fed. We all knew peas and carrots were healthy, but we didn't know the vital role they play in our bodies, that they need to be more than just one small serving on our plates once a day and boiled to death until the nutrients was gone. Actually, eating vegetables was never a problem for me. My parents never had to tell my brother or me to finish our vegetables, because we would eat them faster than they would finish their own. Still, I had no idea taking fried foods and fast food completely out of my life was going to be so mind straining and test my will so much. I'm a human with cravings who was used to ordering what I felt like eating.

At one of my favorite restaurants I used to order a buttery chicken dish with buttery mashed potatoes and—you guessed it—buttery vegetables. In place of that, I now had to order a big salad with balsamic vinaigrette and a side of vegetables. I also ate the darker multigrain bread instead of the white bread. At first I wasn't used to ordering those foods, but I have had no problems with the change and clean my plate every time.

If I feel like French fries, I wait to make them at home. That way I know the potatoes (or sweet potatoes) are baked and not fried. As long as I get to make good food, I am completely fine with this changed diet. I don't ignore my cravings for the foods I used to eat. Instead I make it for myself with healthier ingredients. (At the back of the book is a list of some of the foods in my pantry, with healthy substitutes for less healthy foods.) After I stopped complaining that there was nothing to eat, I could make anything I wanted!

Once I was on this diet, everything about me became clean. My face had always been clear, but since becoming a teen I always had a couple of zits popping up. That ended immediately. It was also easier to have clean thoughts and stay positive without nonorganic, unhealthy food bogging me down. Not to mention my portion sizes shrank. Eating such clean foods nourished my body quicker.

Inside, my body felt clearer than it ever had. I didn't know a healthy diet would have such a cleanup effect on my body, mind, spirit, and overall energy level. If alopecia can't be cured, then that's just alopecia. What I know I can do is eat for my body. This autoimmune disease is in combat mode inside me, affecting my hair. I can focus on growing my hair back from chemicals, or I can stop worrying about my hair and trust that eating clean foods can heal my body completely, and therefore heal my alopecia.

It feels good to have full control over something as big as my health. There is a downside, and that's if I choose to eat poorly. If I eat a slice of cake, I own up to it and then don't have another for a while. I just go back to my routine. Eating something unhealthy doesn't shake my routine: it makes it more livable and real. My outcome is always going to be what I do consistently and repeatedly. What I do every now and then can't shake that. It's ironic that my hair is so thick now; it takes two hours to blow-dry it. I laugh every time I put a brush to my hair because my hair is actually attached! Every 6 weeks I go to the hairdressers to get my hair thinned out. Finding that will inside of me to turn my life around created a big change. My healthy lifestyle is a balance of my mind, diet, movement, and chiropractic. It's the perfect balance, if you ask me. My results are just a positive effect of how health repairs and restores your body completely.

Alopecia put me on a quest. I had to learn that getting what you truly want comes from the will of the spirit and a strong belief system. Alopecia was only a prison if I saw it that way. I kept myself in a mentally draining pattern that revolved around having no hair. I learned that a forward perspective is the key to a successful life of achievements and happiness in any field. As cheesy as it sounds, once I got out of my own head and realized alopecia could move me on to my next chapter in life, I made real progress in building a better life.

If my mind was stuck on the image of me being an ugly bald girl, guess what? Then I was an ugly bald girl. How I perceived myself was all that mattered. Once I accepted that, I could make the first move to overcome this disease. I changed my thoughts from energy draining to life changing. I could finally think clearly and focus on what was really important—my health. And now I have a full head of hair.

Nothing's a big problem for me anymore after alopecia. I appreciate everything, and little things make me really happy. I'm into fashion now and love to dress differently and creatively so that I stand out. When my hair got long enough that I didn't need to wear a hat anymore, it felt so nice not to have to cover my head and hide. Now I love to wear hats, especially on bad hair days. I never thought I'd be saying that! New people that I meet who don't know about my alopecia compliment me on how pretty my hair is. Once a friend even said to me: "Do me a favor, Molly, and never cut your hair." My hair used to be straight, but now it's wavy. I recently had to have my haircut and thinned because it is so thick and was getting so long so quickly.

This book is to help you think about your lifestyle, your routines, and your schedule. Think about your health and really focus on that instead of alopecia. Alopecia was controlling me, but now I control alopecia. Take this book for what it is and let it reflect on your lifestyle.

***

For me, change was good. In fact, change was a remarkable feeling. Not only did I overcome alopecia, making me believe in myself on a fundamental level, but also I found myself again. I never dreamed I could feel this amazing. I truly feel gorgeous. All it took was a change of mind to make a change of life. I'm not saying that's easy, but that's where it starts. I feel accomplished in conquering something so personal that robbed me of my life for quite some time. Nothing beats that. I became my true self.

When I got my hair back, I questioned who I was. I lost my hair when I was twelve years old and shut down for three years. When I reawakened I looked different. I'm older and I'm more feminine. What I learned through all of this was not to try to forget everything that I've experienced, but to embrace it. Our experiences are what make us unique individuals. I wouldn't be writing this book if I wanted to be like everyone else and just forget about the negative things that have happened to me. This is my story, and I'm not going to be ashamed of that. It's taken me some mental recovery to get to this point, but now I can embrace all of me.

Acknowledgments

There are so many people that have educated me in the process of getting my hair back. Internet, books and all forms of educational sources have filled my brain with so much knowledge and gave me confidence that the body should not be underestimated in its power of reversing disease and maintaining health.

The very first person I have to bring acknowledgment to is my mom, Janis Vazquez.
We both went threw this experience together being as close as we are. She even offered to shave her hair off to make me feel better. I remember looking at her saying "Are you crazy?" and we both laughed, but I knew she was serious.

My Dad and Brother, Louis Vazquez Jr., Louis Vazquez Sr.
You never treated me different or looked at me differently. You both stayed on the emotional rollercoaster and after the drop our relationship is so much stronger. Your support taught me about unconditional Love.

My grandparents, cousins and friends at the time were always there. This disease would've eaten me alive if I didn't have you guys. Thank you for all of your emotional support.

Another thank you to my very first chiropractor, Dr. Steve. You and your family taught my family so much about the importance of chiropractic and staying healthy in a busy life. When I came into your office, you and your staff made

it so easy to stay positive during a depressing time of my life.
You're healing a sick, subluxated world with every adjustment.

Elizabeth Barrett, my editor, Thank you. You helped me so much during the process of writing this book.

My Photographer, Dove Shore. I emailed you, told you my story, and a couple of days later I was shooting pictures with you in California
as well as meeting your wife
and dogs.
When I had alopecia I wouldn't allow a camera anywhere near me, who knew all this would take place. Thank you for being apart of my journey of piecing myself and confidence back together. You're amazing at what you do, Lets let the pictures do the talking.

Thank you Sally for helping me get the book out there and for typing the delicious recipes for the cookbook!

WHAT TO EAT

All Fruit
All Leafy Green Vegetables
All Vegetables and Root Vegetables

SWEETENERS
Stevia, Agave, Honey, Yacon Syrup, Raw Honey,
Dates, Date Sugar, Coconut Sugar, Pure Maple
Syrup

BUTTER
Coconut oil, Ghee Butter, (use sparingly)

OIL
Cold-pressed extra-virgin Olive oil, Sunflower oil,
Hemp oil, Flaxseed oil, or other nut/seed oils

CHOCOLATE
Raw Chocolate bar made with natural sweeteners.
Dark Chocolate, unsweetened or no less than 75%
cocoa

BREADCRUMBS
Almond Meal (ground almonds), Ground Nuts
(Walnuts, pistachios, cashews, etc.), or gluten-free
Bread- crumbs

GRAINS
Wild rice, brown rice, quinoa, amaranth, millet,
buckwheat, oats, sorghum, teff

LEGUMES
All Legumes (peas, lentils, beans, cashews)

MILK
Almond milk, rice milk, coconut milk, hemp milk. Any of these milks come in unsweetened and vanilla flavors, or even chocolate flavor.

CHEESE
Goat cheese, vegan gluten-free and dairy-free cheese. (Use all options sparingly)

PEANUT BUTTER
Almond, hazelnut, sunflower seed, pumpkin seed, hemp butter, or other nut/seed butters. If Peanut butter is truly loved, buy wild jungle peanut butter that does not contain aflatoxin.

BREAD
Any gluten free bread, usually found in the freezer section of food stores (I use the brand 'food for life' , there Millet bread is amazing. I also love the brand 'Manna bread')

WRAPS / TORTILLAS
Brown rice wraps and gluten-free tortillas; stone ground corn tortillas ('Food for life' is the brand that I use)

What I do everyday for a delicious non-binding wrap is simply: Lettuce wrap ,collard leaf wrap, or nori sheets (seaweed often used as sushi wraps.

RED MEAT, PORK, HAM, BACON etc.
Organic cage-free chicken and eggs; wild fish, such
as haddock, salmon, tuna, etc.

PASTA / SPAGHETTI
Pastas made from gluten-free grains, quinoa, brown
rice, etc. (Eat moderately, since pasta is still
processed and is a binder to the body.) You can buy
in specialty stores pastas made from from
vegetables or beans (mung bean fettuccine!) Also,
Invest in a spirulizer, which can turn vegetables into
spaghetti! I prefer using zucchini.

CANDY / CANDY BARS
FRUIT! Raw food bars, such as Pure bars and Lara
bars. Trail mix, raisins and other dried fruit can give
you the sweetness you need to satisfy your craving.

SODA
Seltzer water (also known as tonic water or soda
water) Add a little lemon/lime or even some fresh
fruit juice for some real soda, without the syrup!
Kombucha is an amazing soda replacement find it
in your nearest food store.

COFFEE
Herbal or decaffeinated teas

WHAT TO AVOID

White sugar, brown sugar, corn syrup

Breadcrumbs made from gluten

White rice, grains containing gluten
[durum, semolina, bulgur, seitan],

Dairy milk

Butter

Canola oil, vegetable oil, soybean oil

Dairy Cheese

Peanut Butter

Any bread with gluten

Wraps and tortillas made from gluten

White or whole wheat pasta

Red meat, pork, ham, (etc)

Candy bars and everyday sweets

Soda

Coffee, any caffeinated beverage

ALOPECIA
&WELLNESS
RECIPES

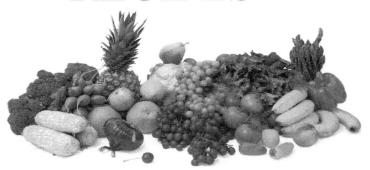

<u>Recipes</u>
Sweet Green Lemonade

1-2 pears or apples
1 head lettuce
4 kale leaves
1 lemon with peel on
Knob of fresh ginger

Juice all ingredients through a juicer (no specific order).

Can't Beet It Juice

1 apple
1 beet
1/2 lime or lemon with peel on
1 head lettuce
4 kale leaves
1/2 cucumber

Juice all ingredients through a juicer (no specific order).

Signature Smoothie

1 1/2 cups cold water
3 ice cubes
2 bananas
1/4 cup hemp seeds
2 handfuls spinach
1 teaspoon maca powder

Blend in blender.

Perfect Pear Smoothie

1 cup cold water
2 pears, chopped
2 handfuls spinach
2 kale leaves
Wedge of lemon, peel cut off
1 tablespoon flax seeds (optional)
3 ice cubes

Blend all ingredients in a blender on high speed, starting with cold water and ending with ice cubes. Makes 24 ounces.

Tinted Green "Cookies and Cream"

1 cup hemp milk, vanilla unsweetened
1/4 cup coconut milk, unsweetened
2 tablespoons raw protein powder, vanilla
1-2 handfuls spinach
1/2 banana (can use frozen)
2 teaspoons almond butter
1 tablespoon cacao nibs (raw crushed chocolate bean)
1 tablespoon coconut oil

Combine liquids in blender with banana. Blend on high speed until smooth. Add rest of ingredients and blend until smooth. Makes 20 ounces.

Sweet Potato Fries

1 sweet potato cut into fries
2 tablespoons melted coconut oil
1/2 teaspoon adobo seasoning
1/2 teaspoon sea salt
1/2 teaspoon coriander
1/2 teaspoon cumin
1/2 teaspoon ginger powder
1/2 teaspoon curry
1/2 teaspoon parsley (dried or fresh)
1/2 teaspoon rosemary (dried or fresh)

Preheat oven or toaster oven to 450 degrees. Place fries in a bowl with coconut oil. Add spices and stir until fries are evenly coated. Place on cookie sheet and bake until desired softness, approximately 10-15 minutes. Serve with ketchup, chipotle mayonnaise, or tahini Caesar dressing.

Mexican Chicken Sausage Stew

2 tablespoons coconut oil
1 large onion, diced
2 carrots, chopped
1 large red bell pepper, diced
2 zucchinis, diced
4 chicken sausages, any flavor (I prefer sundried tomato)

Heat the oil in a large pot and add the next five ingredients. Once the vegetables are soft and the sausage cooked, add:

2 tablespoons tomato paste
32 ounces low sodium chicken broth

1 bunch fresh cilantro, finely chopped
1 tablespoon coriander
2 tablespoons cumin
2 tablespoons chili powder
4 tablespoons coconut cream
3 cups coconut milk
1 teaspoon sea salt
Juice of half a lime

Bring ingredients to a boil and then simmer for 15 minutes. Either allow to thicken for 30 minutes or serve immediately.

Almond Waffles/Pancakes

1 cup almond milk, vanilla flavor
8 eggs, beaten
8 tablespoons coconut oil, melted and cooled
1 teaspoon sea salt
2 tablespoons cinnamon
3 tablespoons honey
4 cups either almond flour, coconut flour, ground flax seed flour meal, or brown rice flour

Mix ingredients in a large bowl. Coat waffle maker with coconut oil (so batter doesn't stick) and add batter to waffle maker. Cook according to manufacturer's instructions. Or oil a griddle with coconut oil and make as pancakes.

Teriyaki Chicken

1 pound chicken pieces, boneless or bone in
1/2 cup coconut aminos (soy substitute)
1/4 cup coconut crystals (sugar substitute)
3 cloves garlic, crushed
1 teaspoon mustard

Place chicken in a plastic bag and pour other ingredients over it. Shake well and marinate at least 3 hours or overnight. The longer the better.

Sweet Lou's Granola Bars

12 fresh dates, seeds removed
1 tablespoon coconut oil
2 cups granola (I use Purely Elizabeth)

Put all ingredients in a food processor and blend together until they form a dough. Oil a 9x9 inch pan and spread the dough in it. Melt 3 ounces of your favorite dark chocolate and pour over the granola dough. Cover with foil and freeze for 3-4 hours to harden the chocolate and dough. Let sit for about 30 minutes before cutting and serving

Peanut Butter Granola Bar

Follow the recipe for Sweet Lou's Granola Bars, but add 4 tablespoons of peanut butter to the food processor.

Cream of Broccoli Soup with Chicken Sausage

4 tablespoons coconut oil
1 onion, chopped
1/2 cup water
Juice of 1 lemon
4 chicken sausages, diced
2 zucchinis, diced
2 1/2 cups broccoli (approximately 2 smaller heads
or 1 large), chopped small
1 green bell pepper, diced
2 cups coconut milk
5 tablespoon creamed coconut
32 ounces low sodium chicken broth

Put onion, water and lemon juice in a food
processor or blender. Blend until somewhat pasty.
Melt 2 tablespoons of the coconut oil in a large pot
and add the onion paste. Bring to a boil and lower
the heat to medium. Add spices: 1 teaspoon each of
paprika, sea salt, garlic powder, dried dill, dried
parsley, mustard powder, sage; 1 tablespoon of
turmeric; and a dash of allspice and black pepper.

Veggie and Brown Rice Stir Fry

1 tablespoon olive oil or coconut oil
1 1/2 cooked brown rice
2 carrots, sliced
1 cup broccoli, chopped
1/2 red bell pepper, chopped
1/2 onion, chopped
2 teaspoons brown rice vinegar
2 teaspoons toasted sesame oil
1 teaspoon red pepper flakes or Szechuan pepper

Heat the oil in a frying pan and add all ingredients.
Stir until vegetables are just cooked. Serves one.

Egg White Scramble

1 tablespoon coconut oil or olive oil
4 egg whites
1/4 cup coconut milk, rice milk, or nut milk
Handful chopped spinach
1/2 tomato, diced
Adobo seasoning to taste

In a bowl whisk the eggs white and milk together.
Heat oil in a frying pan and pour in egg mix.
Scramble the eggs by "sweeping" the eggs with
your spatula. When half cooked, add the remaining
ingredients. Serves one.

Vanilla Nut Crunch Cereal

1/4 cup whole almonds and pistachios
1/4 cups sunflower seeds, pumpkin seeds, and flax
seeds
2 tablespoons agave or pure maple syrup
1 1/2 tablespoons coconut oil, melted
2 tablespoons vanilla (powder or extract)
1 teaspoon almond extract
1 teaspoon coconut extract
1 teaspoon cinnamon
1 handful of shredded coconut
3/4 cup slivered almonds
1/2 teaspoon maca powder

Preheat oven to 350 degrees. Place all ingredients in
food processor. Blend until nuts are small pieces.
Spread onto a baking sheet and bake until nuts are
golden.

Spinach, Goat Cheese, and Tomato Egg White Omelet

1 tomato, diced
1 tablespoon olive oil
1/2 teaspoon sea salt
1/2 teaspoon black pepper
1/2 teaspoon garlic powder

Place ingredients in bowl, mix together, and let sit while making the omelet.

3 egg whites
1/4 cup coconut milk
Handful chopped spinach
2 tablespoons goat cheese
Pinch sea salt
Pinch black pepper
Pinch garlic powder

Whisk egg whites and coconut milk together in a bowl. Heat small frying pan and add olive oil. Add the egg mix. Once the egg mix is half cooked, add the spinach, goat cheese, and spices. Fold the omelet into a half moon and slide onto plate. Either put the tomato mixture over the omelet uncooked (which is really delicious) or quickly heat the tomato mixture in the pan first. Garnish with fresh basil (optional). Serves one.

Carrot Banana Muffins

2 cups almond flour
2 teaspoons baking soda
1 teaspoon sea salt
1 tablespoon cinnamon
1 cup dates
3 ripe bananas
3 eggs
1 teaspoon apple cider vinegar
1/4 cup coconut oil
1 1/2 cups carrots, shredded
3/4 cups pecans, chopped fine

Preheat oven to 350 degrees. In a bowl combine the flour, baking soda, salt, and cinnamon. In a food processor combine the dates, bananas, eggs, vinegar, and oil and blend. Transfer this mixture to a large bowl. Blend in the dry ingredients until evenly combined. Fold in carrots and pecans. Spoon batter into paper-lined muffin tins. Bake for 25 minutes.

Sweet Potato Soup

1 sweet potato, peeled and chopped
1 small onion, chopped
1 zucchini, chopped
3 kale leaves
1/2 teaspoon curry powder
1/2 teaspoon adobo seasoning or garlic powder
1/2 teaspoon coconut oil, melted, or olive oil
3 teaspoons sea salt

In a pot, boil the sweet potato, onion, and sea salt.
Cook for 15-20 minutes. Add zucchini and cook an
additional five minutes. Puree all ingredients in a
blender, including the water the vegetables cooked
in. Toss in the kale, oil, adobo, and curry powder.
Serve topped with your favorite seeds or fresh
herbs. Makes 4 servings.

Light Chicken Piccata

1 skinless, boneless chicken breast, cut in half
lengthwise
Brown rice flour for dredging
Pinch of sea salt and black pepper
3 tablespoons coconut oil
2 1/2 tablespoons olive oil
8 tablespoons fresh lemon juice
1/4 cup chicken stock
1/6 cup capers, rinsed
1/6 cup fresh parsley, chopped

Dredge the chicken in the flour seasoned with salt
and pepper. Shake off excess. In a frying pan over
medium heat, melt 1 tablespoon coconut oil with
the olive oil. When hot, add the chicken and cook
for about 2-3 minutes, until browned. Flip and
brown the other side. Remove chicken. Add to the
pan lemon juice, chicken stock, and capers. Bring to
a boil. As you stir, be sure to scrap up any brown
bits from the chicken—that's where the flavor is!
Add the other 2 tablespoons of coconut oil and
whisk until the coconut oil is completely melted.
Pour over chicken and garnish with parsley. Makes
2 servings.

Quick Flatbread Pizzas

1 frozen brown rice pizza crust or brown rice wrap
Premade pizza sauce
Your favorite toppings

Crisp the crust in an oven or toaster over at 425
degrees. Once it's somewhat crunchy, add the sauce
and your topping.

I usually eat with a salad with balsamic dressing.
Sometimes I put the salad right on the pizza. My
favorite pizza toppings are: pesto sauce, shitake
mushrooms, and arugula or spinach, with a lemon
herb dressing or red onion vinaigrette.

Balsamic Dijon Dressing

3 tablespoons balsamic vinegar
2 tablespoons lemon juice
1 tablespoon Dijon mustard
2 cloves garlic, minced
1/2 cup olive oil

Whisk first 4 ingredients in a bowl to blend.
Gradually whisk in oil. Season with salt and pepper
to taste.

Chia Chocolate Pudding

12 ounces coconut milk, vanilla, unsweetened
1/2 cup raw cacao powder
2 drops chocolate stevia or agave
5 teaspoons almond butter
1 tablespoon chia seeds

In a blender, blend all ingredients in order. Pour into individual serving bowls, if desired, and chill.

Oatmeal Raisin Cookies

1 cup organic rolled oats
1 cup oat or brown rice flour
1 cup almond meal (ground almonds)
1/4 cup shredded coconut (optional but it adds fantastic flavor)
1/2 teaspoon salt
1/4 cup raisins
1/2 cup agave nectar or pure maple syrup
1/2 cup coconut oil, melted
1/2 teaspoon vanilla

Preheat oven to 350 degrees. Mix all dry ingredients together in a large bowl. Mix the remaining ingredients and stir into the dry ingredients with a wooden spoon. Form 1-inch balls and place on an oiled cookie sheet, pressing the balls down with your fingers. Bake for 15-20 minutes. Makes 24 cookies.

For more information on cookbooks, videos, connecting with Molly and for a special Guide to your new healthy lifestyle to make it easier to stay on your new journey (see the password on the next page)

Please Visit Alopecia & Wellness' Website:

www.alopeciaandwellness.com

Here is the special password that will give you

inside access to upload *Diet Guidelines for*

Healing which you can conveniently print out

to take with you grocery shopping & to post

on your refrigerator.

Password: itisuptome